EFT Tapping

Quick and Simple Exercises to De-Stress, Re-Energize and Overcome Emotional Problems Using Emotional Freedom Technique

By

Mike Moreland

Copyright © 2014 Mike Moreland

All rights reserved. No part of this publication may be reproduced, distributed or transmitted in any form or by any means, including photocopying, recording, or other electronic or mechanical methods, without the prior written permission of the publisher, except in the case of brief quotations embodied in reviews.

This book is not intended as a substitute for the medical advice of physicians. The reader should regularly consult a physician in matters relating to his/her health and particularly with respect to any symptoms that may require diagnosis or medical attention. Neither the author nor the publisher assumes any responsibility or liability whatsoever on the behalf of the purchaser or reader of these materials.

ISBN: 1500955485

ISBN-13: 978-1500955489

Table of Contents

Introduction 1

What is EFT? 3
How It All Started..3
EFT versus Acupuncture...5

How Does EFT Tapping Work? 8
The Basic Recipe for EFT Tapping 10
   Step 1: Identify the Issue 10
   Step 2: Rate the Issue 11
   Step 3: Set-Up 12
   Step 4: Tapping Sequence 14
   Step 5: Tune In and Re-rate 19
The 5 Steps of EFT...20

The EFT Heart and Soul Tapping Sequence 22
What Makes This Tapping Sequence Different? 22
How the EFT Heart and Soul Tapping Sequence Is Done..26

EFT Tapping for Stress Relief 29
How Does EFT Work for Stress Relief?...................29
Tapping Sequence and Tapping Statements for Stress Relief..31

Table of Contents

EFT Tapping to Gain Energy 39
How Does EFT Work for Overcoming Fatigue? 39
Tapping Sequence and Statements for Energy 42

Overcoming Emotional Problems with EFT 44
Can EFT Work with Painful Traumas? 45
Tapping Sequence and Statements for Overcoming Emotional Issues 46

More EFT Tips 52

EFT Videos and Other Resources 55
EFT Videos 55
Websites on EFT 55
Books on EFT 56

Conclusion 57

Introduction

Think of everything as energy. Emotions and thoughts are energy. And energy also possesses physical manifestations that are very real.

As we feel a negative emotion, face a traumatic experience, or are pitted against an unfavorable and unpleasant situation, an excess in energy is created. When this excess is not addressed properly, over time, it can result in more serious problems. That is where Emotional Freedom Technique can help.

What is EFT exactly?

Developed by Gary Craig, Emotional Freedom Technique is a psychological acupressure technique that involves tapping near the end points of energy meridians in your body. It is an effective combination of mind-body medicine and acupressure that can help with physical, mental, and emotional health issues. EFT is based on the premise that when we are free from emotional disturbances, we are more likely to be healthy and happy.

EFT has been proven through numerous research studies and by countless practitioners to be highly effective for many issues, including:

- stress
- fatigue, and

Introduction

- emotional problems such as low self-esteem, depression and anxiety

And best of all, EFT is a simple self-help technique that is easy to learn and do on your own. It's no problem to fit EFT into a busy schedule; an EFT session doesn't take long and you can already feel better after just a few minutes.

In this book, you will find all the information you need to learn and use this powerful self-help tool. Millions of people around the world already use EFT for a happier, healthier, and more balanced life. I hope it will do the same for you!

What is EFT?

Also called EFT Tapping or simply Tapping, Emotional Freedom Technique is a healing tool meant to treat emotional, physical, and performance issues. It is based on the premise that unresolved emotional issues stand in the way of improvement involving any aspect of your life. The human body possesses a natural healing potential but emotional stress of any kind may impede it.

There are cases when EFT can work to relieve people of physical symptoms without the need to explore the emotional factors involved in the condition. But longer lasting and more powerful results can be achieved when the related emotional issues are addressed too.

EFT can help you clear out traumas. And with ongoing use of this technique, you may learn and earn a healthy and productive attitude that allows you to welcome any challenges you may face in life.

How It All Started

Before EFT, there was TFT, or Thought Field Therapy, developed by Dr. Roger Callahan, who was a clinical psychologist. Dr. Callahan has dedicated more than 40 years of his life to find ways to heal phobias, trauma, anxiety, addictions, and stress disorders. He himself had suffered from fears and phobias since his childhood.

EFT Tapping

Legend has it that TFT started with one of Dr. Callahan's patients, Mary. Mary had a severe phobia of water. She found it hard to even take a bath. Water caused her a great deal of distress, feeling like water could kill her. Dr. Callahan had been on Mary's case for 18 months. During that time, they tried different therapeutic approaches, such as rational-emotive therapy, hypnosis, and systematic desensitization. All to no avail; Mary continued to be distressed by water and kept having nightmares.

In one of their private sessions, Mary was complaining about a stomachache. Dr. Callahan thought about using a tapping technique to relieve the pain in her stomach. And so he guided her into tapping the area where the stomach meridian begins (under the eye). Surprisingly, Mary was relieved not only of the pain in her stomach, but freed from her phobia as well. To put it to the test, Dr. Callahan guided Mary to the swimming pool, where she didn't show signs of her phobia anymore. In fact, she almost wanted to dive right in, but because she did not know how to swim, she only touched the water and splashed some on her face.

Dr. Callahan used Mary's case to develop Thought Field Therapy in the 80's. The technique involves a set of "algorithms" to tap on specific acupuncture points. Each algorithm is meant to treat specific dysfunctions and ailments. There are many different algorithms that can be used with this technique and Dr. Callahan was generous enough to share and teach them to others.

Among Dr. Callahan's students was Gary Craig, who attended TFT training in 1991. Gary is an engineer from Stanford University who initially pursued a career in insurance sales. Aside from being an engineer, Gary had a particular interest in the field of self-improvement. He started to research this field at a very early age and at one point decided to leave his insurance sales career for what it was and dedicate his life to researching and teaching self-improvement and personal development.

Gary Craig presented in seminars and shared his work through personal performance coaching but he continued to search for better techniques and methods for personal development. And that was when he met Dr. Callahan.

Being introduced to TFT, Gary Craig started to apply the methods on his clients. While taking from Dr. Callahan's technique, Craig also worked to infuse his own methods and simplify the TFT method further. In 1995, Gary Craig released his first training video set, which he called "The EFT Course".

EFT versus Acupuncture

Around 5,000 years ago, the Chinese made a discovery regarding a complex system involving energy circuits running throughout the body. These energy circuits are referred to as meridians. These so-called meridians are the focus of Eastern health practices and lay the foundation for modern day acupressure, acupuncture, and other forms of healing techniques.

EFT Tapping

The energy circuits in your body can't be seen with the naked eye. But even though you can't directly see the energy flowing, you know it's there by its effects, much like the energy in a television set. The energy flowing inside the TV is not visible to the eye, but is apparent through its effects, i.e. the sound and picture it gives.

EFT works in a similar way. You may not see it, but you are able to *feel* the energy flowing within your body. This becomes apparent as you tap near the end points of energy meridians in your body. Through tapping, you can feel the deep changes that occur both in your physical and emotional health. In sum, that is exactly what EFT Tapping is about.

Western medical science focuses on the chemical nature of the human body. Until recent years, modern medical science did not recognize the subtle, yet powerful energy flows that occur within and throughout the body. Over the years, however, this concept has become a popular subject of modern research.

The foundation of EFT is a combination of mind-body medicine and acupuncture. It is important to note that both are backed up by decades of scientific studies. In fact, even prestigious institutions including Harvard and Stanford, among other universities, hospitals, and clinics, recognize their profound significance and effectiveness. Plenty of scientific studies have been conducted and some are ongoing in an effort to validate the significance of EFT Tapping with regard to healing.

What is EFT?

EFT borrows much of its healing process from the meridian system the Chinese developed thousands of years ago. The difference between EFT and acupuncture, however, is that the latter focuses primarily on treating physical ailments. EFT, on the other hand, does not concentrate solely on physical ailments, but addresses and relieves emotional problems as well.

In other words, EFT combines the cognitive benefits of conventional therapy with the physical benefits of acupuncture. The result is a more complete treatment of both physical and emotional issues. It can be said, then, that EFT is the emotional version of acupuncture. The main difference between the two is that EFT does not involve the use of needles.

Rather than using needles, EFT makes use of two basic processes. First is the process of mentally "tuning in" to the specific issues and individual experiences. And the other is the process of stimulating specific meridian points throughout the body. This is done by tapping on these points with the fingertips. If EFT is properly administered and applied, it may help balance out energy flow and clear out disturbances in the meridian system.

How Does EFT Tapping Work?

When there is a disruption in the energy system of your body, you are likely to suffer from negative emotions. Likewise, when you experience a negative emotion, it leads to energy changes. This is why when you are upset, you will feel sluggish too and all kinds of other negative emotions come into play. EFT works by tapping away negative energy blockages and disturbances. It thereby helps restore your energy flow in its natural balanced state, which is ideal for overall health and well-being.

Through EFT, you may experience a change in the way you feel about experiences and situations that initially upset you in the past. As you tap certain points on your body that are equivalent to a specific energy meridian, words will flow easily. This represents the release of negative feelings that haunt and torment you. These can be emotions that you have been holding on to for a long time.

EFT Tapping works by letting your body know which specific experience or issue you would like to work on. EFT is simple, but its simplicity does not take away from its effectiveness. As long as you are clear and specific about the issue, and provided that you handle it properly, you can expel the negativity that holds you back.

The EFT process combines tapping of the energy meridians with voicing of positive affirmations. This

How Does EFT Tapping Work?

combination is effective in clearing emotional blockages that disrupt the body's bio-energy system. As a result, the energy balance in both your mind and body is restored. This makes EFT a crucial element in the achievement of optimal health.

EFT has been proven to help in the process of overcoming stress, fatigue and emotional distress, among many other issues. It is a learnable self-help tool for resolving major issues that hurt us mentally, emotionally, as well as physically.

EFT is quite easy to learn and even beginners can quickly achieve favorable results with tapping. It is a safe, gentle, and non-invasive technique that does not have any side effects. Moreover, you can do it anytime and anywhere you are.

As a self-help tool, the results of EFT sessions may vary from one individual to another. Also, keep in mind that some of your emotional issues may be connected to external factors you can't change, such as the circumstances or people around you. Although you may not be able to fully control these factors, you can, however, use EFT to adjust your response to these external elements, which, in itself, can already be very helpful.

Although supporters claim that EFT has worked where other methods and conventional therapies have failed – like in treating phobias, addiction, etc. – it is important to point out that EFT is not a cure-all. In many cases, EFT has also worked in relieving physical pain. But this technique should never be used in place of medical treatment. For serious illnesses, always consult a doctor.

The Basic Recipe for EFT Tapping

The founder of Emotional Freedom Technique, Gary Craig, developed a Basic Recipe for the application of EFT Tapping. This recipe involves five basic steps:

- Step 1: Identifying the issue
- Step 2: Rating the issue
- Step 3: The set-up
- Step 4: The tapping sequence
- Step 5: Tuning in for re-rating

Step 1: Identify the Issue

The first step involves identifying the issue, problem, or emotion you want to work on. What is troubling you? Use it as the target to be addressed during the tapping session. You have to give it a name. For instance, if you are struggling with a bad temper, state it this way: *"I find it difficult to control my temper."*

By assigning a name to the issue, you focus and turn your attention to it, along with the energy disruptions this issue creates. For the EFT session to be effective, you must target one issue at a time.

How Does EFT Tapping Work?

Now, if you find it tough to tune in to the issue, or if it is too painful to think about, it may be a better idea to seek professional help rather than performing EFT as a self-help tool. If you are dealing with a particularly difficult issue such as depression, it is important to go through the issue one layer at a time.

Work on the surrounding issues first before diving in deep to the problem. Don't start with emotional issues that are too threatening to handle on your own. It may hurt more than it helps.

Step 2: Rate the Issue

After identifying the issue you want to work on, it is important to rate the problem. Rate it on a scale from 0-10 with 0 as no problem whatsoever and 10 as the worst. This rating serves as a comparison for how you feel about the issue before and after the tapping rounds. It serves as a measure of how helpful EFT is to your case.

When dealing with emotional issues, founder Gary Craig recommends that you re-live the memories and replay them in your mind to help you assess the discomfort or displeasure you feel about this issue.

When rating the issue at hand, it is helpful to ask questions. How intense is the displeasure you feel as a result of the issue on a scale from 0-10? How upset does it make you feel to think about the issue? How much do you want to work or resolve this matter? How anxious does it make you feel? These kinds of

EFT Tapping

questions will help you further in placing the issue on the intensity scale.

Step 3: Set-Up

To do the set-up, you first need to come up with a statement that focuses on the issue you want to resolve. Through the set-up statement, you must acknowledge the issue. At the same time, the statement must be followed by a self-affirming phrase. With this structure, you involve exposure therapy and cognitive therapy at the same time, by tuning in to the issue and voicing out positive affirmations about the specific problem you are dealing with.

The basic structure of the set-up statement goes something like this:

> *"Even though _____ (state the identified issue), I deeply and completely accept myself."*

Here are a few examples of set-up statements:

> *"Even though I have trouble controlling my temper, I deeply and completely accept myself."*
>
> *"Even though I find it hard to fall asleep, I deeply and completely accept myself."*
>
> *"Even though I am stressed about work, I deeply and completely accept myself."*
>
> *"Even though I find it hard to connect with my family, I deeply and completely accept myself."*

How Does EFT Tapping Work?

"Even though I am often irritated with my spouse, I deeply and completely accept myself."

As you tune in to the issue and focus on the problem, you may find it difficult to believe in the affirmation. Nevertheless, these affirmations are important, as they help in developing self-acceptance. They are instrumental in the process of learning to accept yourself for all that you are. Even though saying the statements repeatedly is sufficient, preferably say them with conviction if you can.

The set-up statement is meant to allow the emotion to simply be, free from resistance and rejection of oneself. The self-acceptance phrase with the process of tuning in and rating the intensity of the issue brings it to the present moment. It makes the issue and the emotion real.

With this structure of the EFT process, the emotion can be expressed and felt in a safe manner. That is because a clear distinction is made between the unacceptability of the issue and the complete and unconditional acceptance of oneself.

In the set-up phase, you use only *one* tapping point. This is the **karate chop point**, the part of the hand that is used for making karate chops. It is the fleshy part on the outer side of your palm, between the wrist and the baby finger.

Say the set-up statement aloud while gently tapping (with two or more fingers) on the karate chop point of

EFT Tapping

your hand. If you can't say the statement out loud because you are in the company of others, it is enough to say the words silently to yourself.

Repeat the set-up statement **at least three times** while you keep tapping the karate chop point. You can stop after three repetitions, but you are free to continue until you feel completely comfortable. Do you feel relaxed and ready to continue? Then let's move on to step 4!

Step 4: Tapping Sequence

After finishing the set-up phase, we'll start with the tapping sequence. We are going to tap on the following eight key meridian points:

1. Start of the Eyebrow – Between the top of the nose and the start of the eyebrow.

2. Side of the Eye – The bony part on the outside of your eye, near your temple.

3. Under the Eye – The bone underneath the eye, on the top of the cheek.

4. Under the Nose – Between your nose and your upper lip.

5. Chin – The indentation found between your lower lip and your chin.

How Does EFT Tapping Work?

6. Under the Collarbone – Right under the collarbone, about two inches from the midpoint of your body.

7. Under the Arm – Found on the side of your body, this meridian point lies approximately four inches below your armpit. It is on the same level as the nipple for men. And for women, it is in the middle of the bra strap.

8. Top of the Head – The highest point on the top of your head.

For better reference, please refer to the diagram below.

EFT Tapping

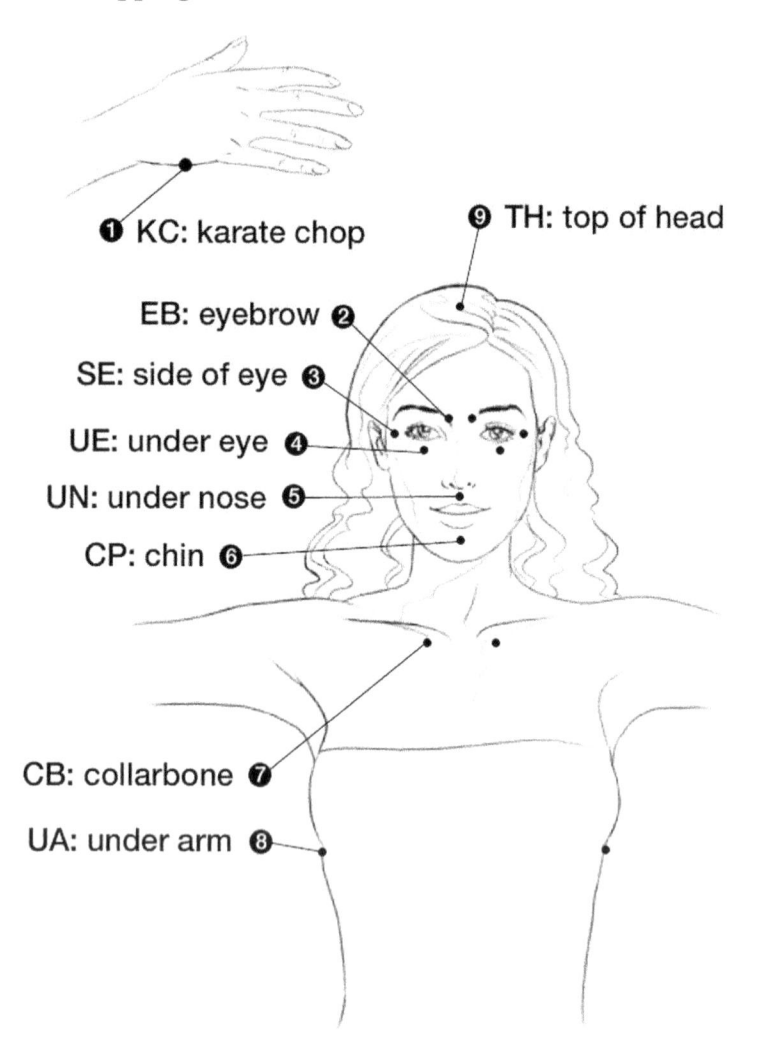

- ❶ KC: karate chop
- ❷ EB: eyebrow
- ❸ SE: side of eye
- ❹ UE: under eye
- ❺ UN: under nose
- ❻ CP: chin
- ❼ CB: collarbone
- ❽ UA: under arm
- ❾ TH: top of head

As you can see in the diagram, some of the tapping points are mirrored on both sides of the body. It does not matter whether you tap on the left or right side of the body, as long as you keep it consistent.

To achieve the right tapping technique, apply firm but gentle pressure. Do it as like you are drumming the

How Does EFT Tapping Work?

tips of your fingers on a desk. Remember to use the tips of your fingers and not your nails. When tapping on the three wider areas, i.e. the collarbone, top of the head, and under the arm, you can use two or more fingers, according to your own preference. However, when tapping the other meridian points, it is important that you only use two fingers, preferably the middle and index finger. This is because these tapping points are smaller and more sensitive areas.

Tap each meridian point in the stated sequence, starting with the inside of your eyebrow and ending on the top of your head. By tapping these points, you work on stimulating your body's energy system, thereby encouraging harmony and balance.

But tapping alone is not enough, it is also important that you speak out a **reminder phrase**. This phrase states the issue at hand. It is the first and negative portion of your set-up statement. For instance, if your set-up statement is *"Even though I find it tough to control my temper, I deeply and completely accept myself,"* then your reminder phrase is *"I find it tough to control my temper."* You can also just say *"I feel _____ (state the emotion, issue or problem)."*

The purpose of this phrase is to keep your focus on the issue at hand. Conventional therapies avoid negative statements. EFT, on the other hand, considers the focus on the negative as an essential part in releasing the issue, problem, or negative emotion.

EFT Tapping

The tapping sequence, however, should not *end* with negative phrases alone. The **second and subsequent** rounds of tapping should highlight **positive** affirmations, suggesting you can overcome the issue.

For the second and subsequent tapping rounds, speak one positive phrase as you tap each meridian point. Below are a few samples you can refer to.

"I believe in my ability to change and solve this issue."

"I am pleased knowing that I can feel calm about this emotion."

"I feel joy about these positive changes."

"I am choosing to feel relaxed despite this issue."

"I am happy because I feel like I am accomplishing so much."

"It feels good to be free from this negative emotion."

"I enjoy the peace and calm I have right now."

"I love knowing I have found a solution to my problem."

"I love, respect, and appreciate the person that I am."

"I am more relaxed and joyful now."

"I am choosing to let go of my negative emotions."

Always speak out loud when you're tapping, as this will keep your mind focused on the issue. In public places or around company, just say the words silently to yourself.

It is up to you how many rounds of tapping you do in your EFT session. Keep tapping until you feel more relaxed.

Step 5: Tune In and Re-rate

For the final part of the EFT exercise, you will be asked to revisit the issue. Tune in to how you are feeling about it after the tapping session. Rate it from 0-10.

Do you still feel the same intensity? Does the issue still make you feel upset as much? Do you still feel the same level of anxiousness thinking about it? Assess how you feel about it now and go back to your rating in Step 1. Is there any difference?

If you feel you haven't reached the result you're looking for, continue tapping. Simply go back to the set-up phase in Step 3 and start tapping again from there. Update your set-up statement based on how you're feeling now, for example saying something like *"I release this remaining stress."*

You can keep tapping until:

- the intensity of your issue reaches 0, or
- the intensity of your issue stops reducing

EFT Tapping

In some cases, repeated and continuous tapping may be necessary, especially when it comes to deep seated emotional issues. If there are no significant changes, improve your methods. Try out different things. Improve your phrases. Relax and focus more. But if you feel like the issue does not further improve or is satisfactorily resolved, you can stop tapping on the issue and move on to other things you want to work on.

The 5 Steps of EFT

To summarize, here are the 5 basic steps for EFT tapping:

Step 1: Identify the issue – Tune in and identify your issue, problem, or emotion.

Step 2: Rate the issue – What is the level of intensity of your issue? Rate it on a scale from 0 to 10 with 0 as no problem whatsoever and 10 as the worst.

Step 3: Set-up – Based on the issue you want to resolve, come up with a set-up statement with the following structure: *"Even though _____ (state the identified issue), I deeply and completely accept myself."* Keep tapping the karate chop point on the outer side of your palm while saying your set-up statement aloud at least three times.

Step 4: Tapping sequence – Tap on the eight meridian points in the recommended sequence, while saying your reminder phrase out loud. For the first tapping round, use your issue as your reminder phrase. For example: *"I feel very stressed out."* For the second and subsequent rounds of tapping, say statements in the form of positive affirmations, suggesting you can overcome the issue. For example: *"I choose to feel calm and relaxed."*

Step 5: Tune in and re-rate – Tune in and rate your issue again on a scale from 0 to 10. If necessary, go back to step 3 and continue tapping. Update your set-up statement based on how you're feeling now. Keep tapping until the intensity of the issue reaches 0 or stops reducing.

The EFT Heart and Soul Tapping Sequence

In addition to the classic EFT protocol described in the previous chapter, there is another tapping sequence referred to as the **EFT Heart and Soul tapping sequence**.

The Heart and Soul tapping sequence is an excellent alternative and just as easy to use as the classic EFT tapping sequence presented in the previous chapter. I'd recommend giving both a try to see which one you find most comfortable and effective.

What Makes This Tapping Sequence Different?

According to Dr. Silvia Hartmann, author of *Energy EFT*, Emotional Freedom Technique is essentially energy work. It is not just about tapping or touching points. The conscious mind plays a special role in this energy work. In fact, the mind has a huge impact on whether or not an EFT session works. If you unconditionally embrace the concept that EFT is about working with energy, a better result from EFT can be achieved. Otherwise, practical blockages may occur.

The Heart and Soul protocol was developed in an effort to address these possible practical blockages that may disrupt a smooth flow of energy. When such disturbances are eliminated, every single round of tapping can produce the best results. It will lead to a

The EFT Heart and Soul Tapping Sequence

maximum increase in energy flow. As a matter of fact, this protocol or tapping sequence was designed with energy at the center.

There are seven main differences between the Heart and Soul protocol and the classic EFT protocol:

1. Heart Healing Posture

You start the Heart and Soul tapping sequence by putting both your hands on the center of your chest. This posture helps you connect with the center of your body's energy system. This way, you can speak your set-up statement in a more mindful and focused manner. It is particularly helpful if you are performing EFT with a healing intention.

The heart healing posture is also done at the end of the tapping sequence with the intention of bringing more focus on the treatment and ending it with the practitioner feeling centered and grounded. It also encourages cognitive insights, which can be very valuable.

2. Top of the Head

The crown point consists of various energy entrances and exits. It serves as the central power channel of the body's energy system. This point is especially effective in treating different kinds of addictions and as a real power point of energy, it can help with many other things as well.

EFT Tapping

The classic protocol also taps on the crown point, but the difference is that instead of ending with the crown point, the Heart and Soul tapping sequence puts it at the beginning. From the top of the head, everything moves down the body to other treatment points, following gravity. Because of this, some practitioners believe this sequence to be more natural.

3. Third Eye Point

The third eye point (the center of the forehead) is left out on the classic protocol. However, it is essential in the Heart and Soul protocol because the third eye point represents global consciousness. It is a representation of spirituality.

Tapping the third eye signifies calling in higher powers for assistance in the process of healing and change, as well as asking our higher selves to be involved and more responsive during the session. Adding this point to the sequence provides a more rounded form of self-healing in EFT.

4. Underarm Point Eliminated

The Heart and Soul tapping sequence drops the underarm point simply because some people may find it off putting or have a hard time locating the exact point to tap on.

5. Finger Points

The Heart and Soul protocol also involves tapping points on all five fingers. These points can allow stuck energy to flow out of the body.

6. Emphasis on Breathing

Breathing is an essential part of the Heart and Soul tapping sequence. It is meant to help release stress and relax the practitioner. The right breathing technique can significantly contribute to the improvement of the energy flow.

The Heart and Soul tapping sequence integrates deep breathing into the exercise not only in the beginning but also throughout the sequence. Taking a nice deep breath as you transition from one point to another can assist in the creation of rhythm, which is stabilizing and helps the flow of energy.

7. Set-Up Statement

For the set-up statement, the phrase *"I deeply and completely accept myself"* is optional. Especially for beginners, this last part of the set-up statement may be difficult if they don't really believe in it and this could reduce the effectiveness of the EFT session.

In the Heart and Soul protocol, it is sufficient to simply state the issue in your own words as succinctly as possible. So if you are dealing with a lot of stress, your set-up statement would simply be something like *"I have a lot of stress."* Giving attention only to the

EFT Tapping

actual problem at hand makes sure that the EFT session remains focused and doesn't get side tracked into other issues.

How the EFT Heart and Soul Tapping Sequence Is Done

0. The Heart Centre – To start the tapping round, assume the heart healing posture. Place both your hands flat on your chest. Take a deep breath in and slowly breathe out. Do this three times.

1. Top of the Head – Speak your set-up statement and begin tapping the crown point. Breathe in and out deeply before moving from one treatment point to another. Repeat your set-up statement at every tapping point.

2. Third Eye Point - This point is located at the center of the forehead.

3. Start of the Eyebrow – Between the top of the nose and the start of the eyebrow.

4. Corner of the Eye – On the bone in the corner of your eye.

5. Under the Eye – On the bone right below your eye, in line with your pupil if you look straight ahead.

6. Under the Nose – Between your nose and your upper lip.

The EFT Heart and Soul Tapping Sequence

7. Under the Mouth – The indentation found between your lower lip and your chin.

8. Under the Collarbone – This point is found in the angle formed by the breastbone and collarbone.

9. Thumb – All finger points are located on the side of the finger, in line with the nail bed.

10. Index Finger

11. Middle Finger

12. Ring Finger

13. Little Finger

14. Karate Chop Point – On the side of your hand.

0. The Heart Center - To end the tapping sequence, return to the heart healing position. Take a few moments of silence for reflection. Breathe in and out three times, deeply and slowly.

Note that you keep repeating the set-up statement at every tapping point. So in this exercise, your reminder phrase is the same as your set-up statement. This ensures that it is at all times clear what issue you're working on. So if your problem is *"I have a lot of stress,"* that will be your set-up statement and reminder phrase all through the session.

The diagram below illustrates all the tapping points of the Heart and Soul protocol.

EFT Tapping

www.1-EFT.com
EFT Heart & Soul by Dr S Hartmann 2010
Based on Classic EFT by Gary Craig 1996

EFT
Emotional
Freedom
Techniques

- Top of the head
- Third Eye point
- Eyebrow point
- Corner of the eye
- Under eye
- Under nose
- Under mouth
- Under Collarbone

Finger Points:
Thumb
Index Finger
Middle Finger
Ring Finger
Little Finger

Karate Chop Point

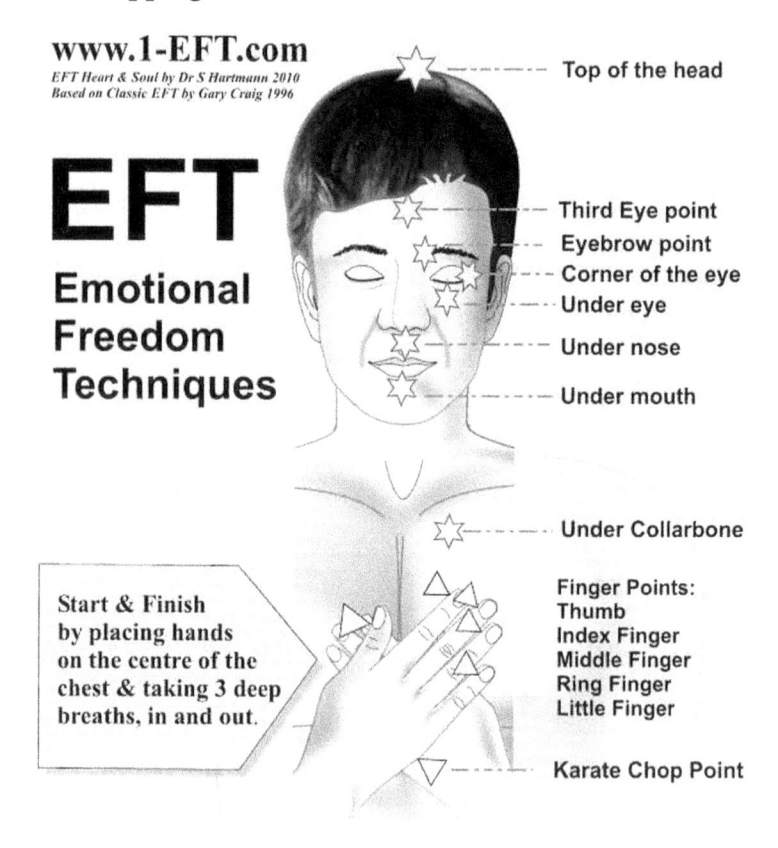

Start & Finish by placing hands on the centre of the chest & taking 3 deep breaths, in and out.

You have now learned how to do EFT Tapping, using either the classic EFT protocol or the Heart and Soul protocol. You can pick the one you find most comfortable and effective, but you can also use them interchangeably if you like.

In the next chapters, we will take a more detailed look at specific issues you may have that you can use EFT for. We will cover EFT for *stress relief, gaining energy,* and *overcoming emotional problems.*

EFT Tapping for Stress Relief

In this fast-paced world, where you constantly have to keep up, stress has become ingrained in our culture. Indeed, stress has become epidemic. What makes stress all the more problematic, is that it is known to cause different types of physical pain, heart disease, premature aging, and other stress-related health conditions. But there are various things you can do to get it out of your system.

Some people do yoga while others do running. Other stress-relieving techniques commonly used include meditation and numerous forms of exercise. Although these stress relieving methods are helpful, the problem with them is that you need to dedicate some time to do them. After all, you cannot pull out a yoga mat during office hours. The good news is that you can also use EFT to effectively relieve your stress. Not only is it quick, but you can also do a tapping session just about whenever and wherever you are.

How Does EFT Work for Stress Relief?

EFT works by reducing the levels of cortisol, the hormone responsible for causing stress. Over a long period of time, when we experience stress, our cortisol levels increase significantly. If this is not addressed properly, it could lead to serious health conditions. But with the help of tapping, we can work on lowering the cortisol levels in our body. This can also help in mitigating our body's response to stress.

EFT Tapping

According to research, EFT is not only effective but its results are also immediate because it combines emotional, mental, and physical stress relief. Dr. Dawson Church, a renowned tapping researcher, points out that by tapping, we send signals bypassing the frontal lobes directly to the mid-brain, where the stress center is. He says EFT works better than talk therapy because it engages both the mind and body. In comparison, EFT is like getting a psychotherapy session and a massage at the same time.

Dr. Dawson conducted a study that involved 83 participants who were divided into three groups. Group 1 received an hour of EFT while Group 2 went through talk therapy for an hour. The third group did not receive any treatment at all. The results were outstanding. The first group who received an EFT session showed 24 percent reduction in their cortisol levels, while the other two groups did not demonstrate any real change. Using the Symptom Assessment-45 (SA-45), which is a standard psychological assessment tool, the EFT group also demonstrated reduced levels of psychological symptoms.

EFT can access the part of the brain responsible for initiating negative reaction to fear, which is also known as "fight or flight" response. This part of the brain is called the amygdala. The ability of EFT to influence the amygdala is what makes EFT Tapping so effective.

Tapping Sequence and Tapping Statements for Stress Relief

For this exercise, we will use the classic EFT protocol. Specific attention will be paid to step 4 of the EFT exercise by presenting a number of stress relieving statements to be used in a series of eight tapping rounds.

Step 1: Identify the Issue

Tune in to the issue and identify it. In this case, you are going to work on your stress.

Step 2: Rate the Issue

Rate your stress on a scale from 0 to 10.

Step 3: Set-Up

Tap your karate chop point on the outer side of your palm and say your set-up statement aloud at least three times. For example: *"Even though I am stressed about work, I deeply and completely accept myself."*

Step 4. Tapping Sequence

For tapping to work, it must be used in combination with focusing phrases to remember the main issue you are working on, which, in this case, is stress. As you focus on the issue and tap on your acupressure points, the energy system that flows within and

EFT Tapping

throughout your body becomes balanced. As a result, you gain emotional relief.

When using focusing phrases to work on relieving stress, you have to be as specific as possible with regard to the reason or source of your stress. For instance, if you are particularly worried about an incoming job interview, you have to state it that way. Keep in mind, the more detailed and specific you are about the issue and its corresponding source or reason, the better.

There are a total of eight rounds here and in the first round, you will start by expressing the feeling of stress you have. The next round involves getting to understand the issue. The third round encourages you to explore possibilities and in the fourth round, you must address the doubts in your mind. The fifth round is meant to relax you a little. The aim of the sixth round of tapping is to give you hope. The seventh round is meant to slow you down. And the final round is where you choose peace and calm.

We are going to use the eight tapping points of the classic EFT protocol: the start of the eyebrow, the side of the eye, under the eye, under the nose, the chin, the collarbone, under the arm, and the top of the head. Here are some statements you could use as you tap the meridian points in the recommended sequence:

Tapping Round 1: Expressing Your Feeling of Stress

Start of the eyebrow: *"There are just so many things I have to do!"*

Side of the eye: *"It is too overwhelming and it stresses me out!"*

Under the eye: *"How am I supposed to do all this work?"*

Under the nose: *"I am tired of having to rush and work frantically to get these things done."*

Chin: *"I have so much pending work and it is hanging over me like a big cloud."*

Collarbone: *"All these tasks loom over me."*

Under the arm: *"I feel the urgency, but to the expense of clarity."*

Top of the head: *"I know I will do much better with clarity."*

Tapping Round 2: Trying to Understand Your Feeling of Stress

Start of the eyebrow: *"I can think clearer and better when I am not in a rush."*

Side of the eye: *"It makes me feel like I am in an emergency room."*

EFT Tapping

Under the eye: *"There is no danger but the sense of urgency is too much for me."*

Under the nose: *"I know this is not a struggle to fight or flight."*

Chin: *"I do understand that some work must be done now."*

Collarbone: *"And there are some tasks that can be done at a later time."*

Under the arm: *"Some of this work needs to be saved for later."*

Top of the head: *"I can separate the tasks that need to be done now from those that can be done later."*

Tapping Round 3: Exploring Possibilities

Start of the eyebrow: *"By putting all the work in a 'do now' pile, I am drowning myself."*

Side of the eye: *"It is nice if everything can just fall into place."*

Under the eye: *"Like how it is in a puzzle."*

Under the nose: *"I think I can work this out."*

Chin: *"Perhaps I can space out some of the work."*

Collarbone: *"That way, it can fit better in the big picture."*

Under the arm: *"That will help me handle things better and more responsibly."*

Top of the head: *"That will make me proud for doing an awesome job."*

Tapping Round 4: Addressing Your Doubts

Start of the eyebrow: *"I do not feel the sense of urgency in my bones."*

Side of the eye: *"I am more likely to slack off."*

Under the eye: *"I am not capable of pushing myself enough."*

Under the nose: *"Do I have to force myself to do more?"*

Chin: *"Could I be holding myself back by resting even for only a few minutes?"*

Collarbone: *"What if I just complete the tasks that I can actually manage?"*

Under the arm: *"That would not overstretch me."*

Top of the head: *"That may not overwhelm me with stress."*

Tapping Round 5: Start to Relax

Start of the eyebrow: *"Doing the tasks I can manage…"*

Side of the eye: *"does not have to overwhelm me."*

Under the eye: *"The pressure to manage everything…"*

EFT Tapping

Under the nose: *"only pushes me down and backwards."*

Chin: *"It does not help drive me toward my goal."*

Collarbone: *"I am smart and I know how to prioritize."*

Under the arm: *"I am choosing to slow down to get my priorities straight and plan my schedule better."*

Top of the head: *"This will help me create a more realistic to-do list."*

Tapping Round 6: Be More Hopeful

Start of the eyebrow: *"It is more helpful than creating mental notes."*

Side of the eye: *"It really does not matter if I work in a frenzy..."*

Under the eye: *"to get more done because tasks do take time to complete."*

Under the nose: *"I may not be able to pull everything off..."*

Chin: *"but that is alright..."*

Collarbone: *"as long as I am doing my best at all times."*

Under the arm: *"Things may just fall into place."*

Top of the head: *"That would be a real treat!"*

Tapping Round 7: Take It Easy and Slow Down

Start of the eyebrow: *"Is it possible to live a full life and not miss a beat?"*

Side of the eye: *"Can I afford to go without feeling the need to rush?"*

Under the eye: *"Is it even healthy to keep on rushing through life?"*

Under the nose: *"I am choosing to take a step back and slow down."*

Chin: *"I will figure it out in no time."*

Collarbone: *"I do not need adrenaline rush for motivation."*

Under the arm: *"I am in control when I am relaxed."*

Top of the head: *"Being calm keeps me in charge."*

Tapping Round 8: Choose Peace and Calm

Start of the eyebrow: *"I choose to let go of nervous energy."*

Side of the eye: *"I choose to complete tasks I can manage now."*

Under the eye: *"I choose to release stress and stop worrying about the future."*

Under the nose: *"I trust myself to do what is needed."*

EFT Tapping

Chin: *"I choose to have clarity."*

Collarbone: *"I choose to take a deep breath and relax."*

Under the arm: *"I choose to feel good about myself because I am competent and responsible."*

Top of the head: *"I choose to be calm and feel confident."*

Step 5. Tune in and re-rate – Tune back in and re-rate your stress level on a scale from 0 to 10. If necessary, go back to step 3 and continue tapping.

EFT Tapping to Gain Energy

Everyday life can be hectic and stressful. When you have a lot of stuff going on, you may find yourself lacking energy and feeling fatigued.

The following EFT tapping sequence is aimed at helping you rebalance your energy system. It will give you a quick energy boost and help you become more alive and alert. If you do this exercise on a daily basis, it will also boost your overall energy level.

How Does EFT Work for Overcoming Fatigue?

To understand how EFT works for overcoming fatigue and gaining energy, it is important to go through the tapping points one by one. For this exercise, we are going to use four tapping points that are directly related to the body's energy system. These are:

1. Under the eyes on the cheekbones

2. The collarbone

3. The thymus point or center of the chest, and

4. The spleen neurolymphatic points

1. Under the Eyes for Staying Grounded and Connected with Your Rhythm

It is society that creates a schedule for us that we have to follow. This allows us to conform but it also goes against our natural rhythm, which stresses and wears us out.

The stomach meridian is the pathway of energy and it flows from around your eyes down the front of your body and legs, all the way down to the second toe. The tapping point affecting the stomach meridian is found under the eyes on the cheekbones.

When the energy flows smoothly in this meridian, you feel much more connected with the energies of the earth. This puts your body in a perfect rhythm. When you tap these acupressure points, your energy becomes more grounded and drives your hormones in support of your body's natural rhythm.

In terms of psycho-energy, when your body is in its natural rhythm, it is able to metabolize better. It also helps you become more adaptable to the things you find hard to adapt to. Reaching your natural rhythm will make you feel more stable and grounded so you can go with the natural flow.

2. The Collarbone for Encouraging a Forward Direction in the Flow of Energy

If you get tired even when you are only walking forward, it is a definite sign that you should pay more attention to these meridian points. These acupressure points are found just below your clavicle or collarbone. To locate them, position the tips of your fingers on the U-shaped notch above your breastbone. Now move your fingertips out on each side and about an inch down. You may feel a small depression here.

This is where the kidney meridians end. The energy pathways of the kidney meridians start under the ball of your foot, moving up the inside of your leg, travelling up the front of your body, and finding its end at your collarbone.

By tapping on these points, which are also known as "K-27 points", you encourage the energy flow to move in a forward direction passing through all your meridians. This helps kick start your energy system, making you feel more energetic and alert.

3. The Thymus or Center of Chest for Gaining Life Energy

Dr. John Diamond, who wrote *Life Energy*, points out that it is the thymus gland that is responsible for controlling the body's life energy. This gland is found right beneath the upper part of your breastbone at the center of the chest. It has a huge role to play in the immune system. This is exactly what Tarzan thumps before he gets an instant boost of energy.

4. The Spleen Neurolymphatic Points for Eliminating Toxins and Assimilating Change

As part of the lymph system, these points assist in flushing out toxins from the body. These points are the depression located between the 7th and 8th rib. It is found right below the level of the sternum or breastbone. To locate these points, move your fingertips beneath your breast in line with the nipples. Then move them further down just over the next rib.

By thumping, not tapping, these points, you can eliminate toxins and regulate hormones and blood chemistry. Performing this exercise also helps with fighting off infections and promoting healthy metabolism of food. It is also known to help relieve stress and dizziness. Moreover, if you want to initiate a change in a specific aspect of your life, the spleen meridian energy is what you need to work on.

Tapping Sequence and Statements for Energy

If you feel any soreness in these points, massage or rub them first before starting with the tapping. As you work on these acupressure points, make sure to breathe in deeply through your nose and breathe out slowly through your mouth. If possible, take three deep breaths as you perform each step. Feel free to do more if necessary.

Under the eyes: *"I am joined with the earth. I feel grounded. I am finding my natural rhythm."*

Take deep breaths. As you tap and repeat these statements, picture the energy travelling from under your eyes to the cheekbones, moving up around your eyes, going to the front of the torso, down to the legs, and ending off the foot right at your second toe.

Collarbone: *"I am balanced and centered. I am gracefully moving forward with my life."*

Visualize the energy flowing from under your foot up to the inside of the legs, travelling further up in front of your body, and ending on the meridian points you are tapping.

Center of the chest: *"My life energy is remarkable. I am filled with love, faith, courage, gratitude, and trust."*

Start by balling up your hand to make a fist. Then, you start thumping the center of your chest like Tarzan does. Take deep breaths and repeat these statements.

Spleen neurolymphatic points: *"Change is always good. I am moving with the flow gracefully."*

Tap beneath the breast in your ribs. Breathe deeply and repeat these tapping statements.

Overcoming Emotional Problems with EFT

EFT can be quite effective in clearing emotional problems and disturbances that may disrupt our meridians. As we face an overwhelming situation, we experience an intense surge of energy that comes in the form of emotions and thoughts coupled by physical sensations that flow through us. Our acupressure points and energy meridians work to transport and grip on the excess energy that is generated as a result. Unfortunately, the energy surge can at times be too much, so that it leads to an overload resulting in a "crash".

With the help of EFT, the excess energy can be released so we can free ourselves from the burden. The excess charge that is trapped in the memory of the cause of the emotional problem, such as a traumatic experience, can be overcome.

EFT tapping acknowledges and addresses negative emotions until they are gradually released. Tapping techniques can be used until excess energy is balanced out. That will help restore the balance in our body's energy system.

To better understand energy disruption, let's use the river analogy. Small avalanches may drive debris into the water. In this case, the current can manage to continue flowing, carrying the debris away. However, if debris is washed into the water continually, the current will not be able to keep up eventually.

Over time, debris can settle and stagnation may occur which will block the flow of the water. As a result, water may back up in certain areas as in the case of excess energy. And in some areas, water may be insufficient. In other words, the river loses balance. This is usually what occurs when you experience stress over a long period of time or are exposed to traumatic experiences without properly addressing them.

Now if the blockages prove to be strong enough, it may even lead to energy reversal. That will cause us to work against ourselves, which is also known as self-sabotage.

Can EFT Work with Painful Traumas?

Human emotions, both positive and negative, are filled with energy. When we allow it, you can feel the "charge" they bring. And in the case of trauma, the "charge" can become too overwhelming.

Conventional therapies are designed to encourage reliving of memories. In this case, a patient is encouraged to submerge himself in the strong currents of pain that remain unreleased. Therapists recommend patients to dive into the deepest parts of their pain, face them, and explore them. To the patient, this is an unpleasant experience to say the least.

EFT Tapping

EFT is unlike conventional therapies in that it does not require an individual to immerse himself in the strong currents of traumatic pain. EFT does not recommend jumping into the deepest part of the pain for the sake of releasing the "charge" of emotions. What EFT does to help with traumatic pain is to reduce its intensity first by addressing the surrounding issue. EFT recommends a step by step process dealing with the surrounding emotions one at a time until the individual is ready to go much deeper. In other words, the EFT approach is comparable to peeling an onion. External issues are addressed first, layer by layer.

Tapping Sequence and Statements for Overcoming Emotional Issues

Overcoming emotional problems is a process. In this section, we will take a look at four tapping rounds, including the specific tapping sequence and statements for overcoming emotional problems.

The first step is recognizing the issue. It is not easy but the only way to work around and overcome the emotional issues that overwhelm you is to recognize and face them.

Now, you have to learn acceptance. To be able to let go and find a resolution for your emotional issues, you have to be able to learn to truly accept yourself, despite of all the issues you are facing. When you resist, change only becomes more difficult. But when you accept yourself unconditionally, you can live freely, free from the shackles of your emotional problems.

As you feel more self-acceptance, the next step is to work on turning things around slowly. When you are accepting yourself more, you learn to open up. This is where possibility statements come into play. They can help in the transformation of negative energy without the subconscious mind locking up. As you open up, you become more relaxed.

The final step involves making a choice. Being open and accepting, your subconscious becomes more welcoming of strong positive affirmations. This is when you make change happen.

We are going to use a new tapping point for this exercise, called the **gamut point**. You can locate the gamut point on the back of your hand by making a fist and drawing an imaginary triangle back from the knuckles of your baby finger and ring finger. The depression in the middle of this triangle is the gamut point.

Tapping Round 1: Recognize and Accept the Issue

Karate chop point: *"I am in pain."*

Top of the head: *"These feelings of hurt overwhelm me."*

Start of the eyebrow: *"My heart is filled with these negative emotions of _____ (be specific)."*

EFT Tapping

Side of the eye: *"I do not know how much of this I can still endure."*

Under the eye: *"It does not seem to stop."*

Under the nose: *"I feel helpless."*

Chin: *"I find it hard to control my emotions."*

Collarbone: *"I do not like feeling this way."*

Under the arm: *"I want to feel better."*

Gamut point: *"I want to let go of the pain."*

All fingers (finger points are located on the side of the finger, in line with the nail bed): *"I want to be happy for a change."*

Tapping Round 2: Learn Self-Acceptance

Karate chop point: *"I acknowledge and accept how I feel."*

Top of the head: *"I embrace who I am."*

Start of the eyebrow: *"Even though I am burdened with these emotions of _____ (be specific), I am still a good person."*

Side of the eye: *"I appreciate myself for being able to endure these challenges all this time."*

Under the eye: *"I am learning to accept, appreciate, and love every aspect of my being."*

Under the nose: *"I am learning to accept myself for everything that I am."*

Chin: *"I appreciate myself for enduring these difficulties."*

Collarbone: *"Despite everything, I am learning and willing to love myself."*

Under the arm: *"I thank, respect, and love myself."*

Gamut point: *"I am open to embracing myself and all parts of me."*

All fingers: *"I accept all of me and everything that I feel."*

Tapping Round 3: Turn the Issue Around

Karate chop point: *"I believe that I will find a way."*

Top of the head: *"I am open to considering different perspectives of this issue (be specific)."*

Start of the eyebrow: *"Perhaps there is another way I have not yet looked into."*

Side of the eye: *"I am feeling that it is possible to put this problem (be specific) behind me."*

Under the eye: *"I am allowing both my mind and body to work this out."*

Under the nose: *"I believe I am capable of letting this go."*

EFT Tapping

Chin: *"I am willing to let changes happen naturally."*

Collarbone: *"I am accepting that I do not have to solve all these problems (be specific) right now."*

Under the arm: *"I am realizing that things will fall into place eventually."*

Gamut point: *"I can find peace."*

All fingers: *"I can let go."*

Tapping Round 4: Let Go and Move Forward

Karate chop point: *"I am choosing to be calm and feel confident."*

Top of the head: *"I have made a decision to let this _____ (be specific) go."*

Start of the eyebrow: *"I choose to be peaceful."*

Side of the eye: *"I take it one day at a time."*

Under the eye: *"I am choosing to heal."*

Under the nose: *"I am reclaiming my personal power."*

Chin: *"I am relaxed. I am choosing to be okay with this _____ (be specific)."*

Collarbone: *"I feel at peace right now."*

Under the arm: *"I am now more open and accepting with this issue (be specific)."*

Gamut point: *"I am reclaiming my personal safety."*

All fingers: *"I am choosing to work this out."*

More EFT Tips

If you've already tried a few EFT sessions, how has it worked out for you so far? Is it living up to your expectations? If it isn't, do not be too quick to blame the method. If tapping does not give the results you're looking for, try the following tips to make the most of EFT.

Add Variety to the Exercise

Do not just get stuck with doing the same sequence and repeating the same statements over and over. If your current method does not work, there is probably something missing or you may be doing something wrong. Find out what it is and make sure to adjust.

It may be tough to figure out what is wrong with the exercises you are doing. But by trying out different things, you should be able to determine which sequence, which statements, and which routines work best for you.

Keep Hydrated

Around 60% of our body consists of water and our brain is even made up of around 75% water. Water is vital to us and without it we wouldn't survive; it flushes waste from our body, regulates body temperature, and delivers nutrients to our cells.

For EFT, it is also important to keep well hydrated. EFT targets electrical energy in the body and water conducts electricity. Practitioners have found that EFT does not give good results when a person is dehydrated. So if tapping does not reduce the intensity of your issue, make sure to drink water before your session. It also helps if you keep some water handy during your sessions so you can keep drinking between tapping rounds.

In general, it is recommended to drink at least 8 glasses of water a day (around 2 liters). Keeping your body well hydrated throughout the day is essential to your health.

Change Your Routine

Are you used to doing EFT during your work break hours in the office? Why don't you change things around a bit and try it out in the morning or as you experience the afternoon slump? The key is not only to try different ways to do tapping, but also to do it in different places and at different times of the day until you find what works best.

Vary the Frequency and Force of Tapping

Try varying the frequency and force of your tapping during sessions. For example, if you are looking for more motivation or energy, tap a bit harder and faster to activate your nervous system more. If, on the other hand, your goal is to feel more relaxed and calm, tap more slowly and deliberately.

EFT Tapping

Use Tapping in Combination with Yoga and Meditation

Yoga and meditation are excellent methods to feel more relaxed and balanced, and they work really well in combination with EFT. Do some light stretching, yoga, or meditation before you start your tapping session. This brings you in the right state of mind and can enhance the effectiveness of EFT. You can also speak your affirmations out loud or mutter them with conviction in between your yoga poses. This combination can help significantly in eliminating emotional stress.

Keep trying new and different things until you find what is right for you!

EFT Videos and Other Resources

Do you want to learn more about Emotional Freedom Technique? By completely grasping the concept of EFT, applying the tapping technique properly, tuning in correctly, and creating specific and appropriate phrases, you should be able to get good results. Below, you can find a few more resources if you want to learn more about EFT.

Use these references to broaden your knowledge and improve your methods. Happy tapping!

EFT Videos

There are many EFT videos on the Internet that you can use to learn more about EFT or improve your tapping skills. What works really well is to watch videos from practitioners demonstrating an EFT session. You can pick a video that focuses on the same issue you want to work on and then just sit back and tap along.

To get started, check out the list of popular EFT videos I've put together on YouTube. Go to www.youtube.com/user/mikemoreland7 and click on the playlist called 'EFT Tapping'.

Websites on EFT

- www.emofree.com
- eft.mercola.com

EFT Tapping

- www.eftuniverse.com
- www.energyeft.com

Books on EFT

- Colin G Smith, *EFT Tapping: How To Relieve Stress And Re-Energise Rapidly Using The Emotional Freedom Technique.*

- Rockride Press, *EFT and Tapping for Beginners: The Essential EFT Manual to Start Relieving Stress, Losing Weight, and Healing.*

- Silvia Hartmann, *Energy EFT.*

- Marion Jaide, *EFT Tapping Blueprint: A Beginner's Simple Step Plan to Overcome Emotional Problems and Achieve Freedom.*

- Anthony Anholt, *Tapping Scripts for Beginners - EFT tapping scripts for stress management, weight loss, energy healing and more that you can use today!*

- Dawson Church, *The EFT Manual.*

- Nick Ortner, *The Tapping Solution: A Revolutionary System for Stress-Free Living.*

All these books are available on Amazon.

Conclusion

Emotional Freedom Technique has gained a reputation worldwide. Millions of people use EFT for a happier, healthier, and more balanced life. Will EFT tapping live up to its promise for you as well? There is no other way to find out than to give it a try.

Use the information you have learned in this book to improve your condition, resolve any emotional or internal conflicts you may be experiencing or any problems you may be facing. Use it to make your life better. Take advantage of EFT to be more positive and happy!

Finally, if you enjoyed this book, please take a minute to share your thoughts and post a review on Amazon. I would really appreciate it, thank you!